Essential Oils for Kids:

30 Best Recipes For Your Kids' To Be Healthy and Smart

Table of content:

Introduction

Many parents get concerned when it comes to trying something with their kids. They think that it might suit them according to their age but that is not the case with essential oils blend. Essential oils are natural and they heal no matter what your age is. It can be used on the toddlers, infants, kids, adults or any person. They only give positive results whoever uses it and never works against it. You just need to know the right blend and if your child likes it fragrance then you can keep on using it to heal them.

Mostly the toddlers give hard time to the parents so you can use the recipes for them to calm them. Moms do not get time to do the house chores due to which they feel angry and scold their children. You can use these recipes and stay calm by yourself and keep your children calm as well.

The essential oils recipes will help you get rid of crankiness and you will feel relaxed that your kid is playing without disturbing you. You can spend time with your spouse easily when your child is sleeping calmly because of the essential oil massage.

You will see the difference in the environment, as well as the behavior of your kid. Many practitioners use essential oils as a therapy for their patients because of the natural herbs included in it. Anything which is natural will never harm you so get started with the perfect blend recipes of diffusers which can make your house smell beautiful and keep your kids aligned with normal activities with staying calm and easy.

Essential Oils for Kids Health

Essential oils do not have any side or hidden effects. You will be glad to use the oils on your kids because they provide ultimate relief which you may be having a long time. They are natural and do not harm you at all. You only need to know the right blends for the specific thing, and you will see how it heals you perfectly without even knowing it.

Essential oils have played a dynamic role in the history where it used to be set as an example to heal someone through the natural means. The essential oils are extracted from the aroma plants which is why the smell of it is so soothing that you wish to keep on smelling it forever.

Some people have aromas of essential oils in their home to feel better, and it also enhances the mood due to which they have diffusers at home. Here are some of the factors which will make you realize the important of essential oils.

- **Treats Minor Illness for the Kids**

Many people have allergies or some illnesses prolong which becomes a tension for you already. It diffuses the basic illness which you can get on daily routines such as flu, coughing and all. The vapors in the air have the power to make you feel better on your chest and head.

Once you inhale it naturally just like you breathe in the air, it will make you feel okay. You will forget that you have the flu and it will stop. It is only the game of the brain. Once that part is normal, you will normally be functioning too, but if that part is a mess, then there is no way out for you to escape it.

- **Creativity Emerges**

When your brain cells are charged, you are active and working more intelligently, but when you get tired, it gets hard to comprehend anything because of the low functionality.

You can escape such situations by having the essential oils at home. It will make your brain function fast all the time whether you are tired or not. You will be able to focus on the thing which you are working on even if you are tired.

There are some of the oils which help you gain the energy and keep your muscles active. If you use the essential oils regularly, there will be a clear difference between the before and after situation.

- **Brings Calmness to the Kids**

Staying calm sometimes becomes hard, but the essential oil does so. It keeps the kids calm even in the situation where there is a mess, and you can get angry. Sometimes when we are frustrated, we tend to take it out of our friends and family, but with the help of having the essential oils and the beautiful scents around you, you will be calmer than before.

- **Cost –Effective**

Essential oil saves you from a lot of the things which can occur to you if you do not have it. It saves you money, and it is a one-time cost which you will have to bear.

You won't have to pay visits to the doctor because the prior job of the essential oils is to keep you healthy psychologically and physically. That is what it takes if you have just one essential oil and perfect recipes of essential oil to be poured into it.

- **No Mood Swings for Children**

Improving moods is the top most response of the essential oils. They work like magic on kids' mood no matter if they are angry or irritate, it works like anything on them.

It turns the negative emotions into positive ones naturally. You can make the positive environment if your brain is working towards that direction too. You can be a hope to someone as well who is depressed from life. Take out time for your spouse with having the essential oils at home, and you will see how the atmosphere turns romantic like nothing before.

- **Relief of Minor Pains**

When we feel pain anywhere, we tend to panic more than the pain. It is because our brain does not accept that something has happened to the body and we tend to fall weak in a trap of getting emotional.

We lose our mind due to which it gets on our head and tension increases the pain by keeping the muscles stressed. You can also use some of the essential oils as a massage which will heal your muscles of the kids. For a headache, just apply the necessary essential oil, and the scent of it will make you feel better for sure.

- **Sleep Peacefully With Essential Oil Blend**

We all know that if you do not get enough sleep time, then your brain activity tends to slow down over the period no matter how hard you try to stay up. It is beyond a human's capacity to stay up for more than 48 hours continuously.

When you have had a hard day, that is when the essential oil works the best for you. It keeps you calm and makes you sleep within seconds with a deep night sleep. Even if you get like 5 hours of sleep daily and that too deep, it will be enough for you to carry on with the tough days. If you feel like taking the essential oils to your office, you can do that too, and the environment will be so friendly which you will love.

Your kid will love to wake up for school every day because of having such a comfortable environment. Human brains are complicated which is why there are so many problems in the world which cannot be resolved and keeps on exaggerating. Well, get a good night sleep with the application of essential oils, and once you get a hold of it, then it is hard to stop it.

- **Breathing Gets Normal**

If you are someone whose chest gets congested every other day, then the essential oil is best for you. The allergies get eliminate with making you breathe faster and easier than before. You won't be breathing fast once you have inhaled the scents of essential oil or while climbing the stairs too.

Keep the essential oils in your room, and you will see the difference that you do not tend to breathe heavier anymore. Heavy breathing can be dangerous because it indicates a lot of weakness in you. You need to make sure to check with the doctor if it does not fix with the essential oils.

Chapter 1 – Energetic Blends for Your School Going Children

A lot of people go through a lot of problems with their children nowadays without them knowing about it and they get irritated for no reason. There are many causes due to which you can feel tired such as stress, fatigue, hormones, constipation, low sugar level, poor posture, food and much more.

Kids go to school every day and then end up having pains by night. Sometimes you do not get to know which way to go and what to do to get some relief which is why you start giving the medications which are not so recommended for the kids.

You can try the awesome recipes for the school going child who will wake up fresh and stay happy all the time. It is necessary that the kids have their moods happy because then it turns into a frustration and becomes a bad signs for their future. Check out the amazing fragrance blends which can keep your child fresh and going with the daily routine life.

Recipe 01: Roll-On Blend – Sweet Dreams

Ingredients:

- 10 ml roller bottle: 1
- Coconut oil: 2 Teaspoons
- Roman Chamomile Essential Oil: 1 Drop
- Geranium Essential Oil: 1 Drop
- Waterproof Label: 1

Directions:

Add essential oils with coconut oil in the roller bottle. Afterwards, put inside the roller attachment along with its lid. Place the waterproof label and keep away at a safe place.

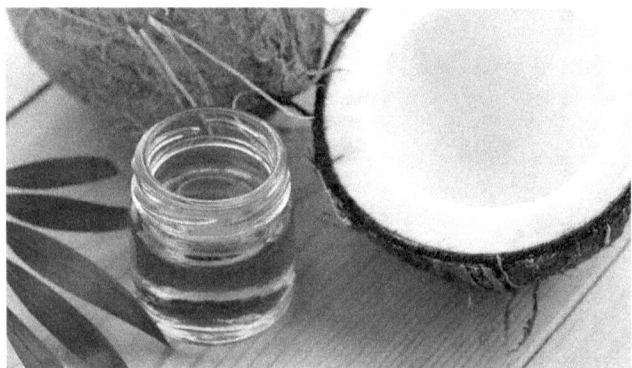

Recipe 02: Roll-on Blend – Mr. Sandman

Ingredients

- 10 ml roller bottle: 1
- Coconut oil: 2 Teaspoons
- Vetiver Essential Oil: 1 Drop
- Royal Sandalwood Essential Oil: 1 Drop
- Waterproof Label: 1

Directions

Add essential oils with coconut oil in the roller bottle. Afterwards, put inside the roller attachment along with its lid. Place the waterproof label and keep away at a safe place.

Recipe 03: Roll-on Blend – Sleepy Head

Ingredients

- 10 ml roller bottle: 1
- Coconut oil: 2 Teaspoons
- Lavender Oil: 1 Drop
- Orange Essential Oil: 1 Drop
- Waterproof Label: 1

Directions

Add essential oils with coconut oil in the roller bottle. Afterwards, put inside the roller attachment along with its lid. Place the waterproof label and keep away at a safe place.

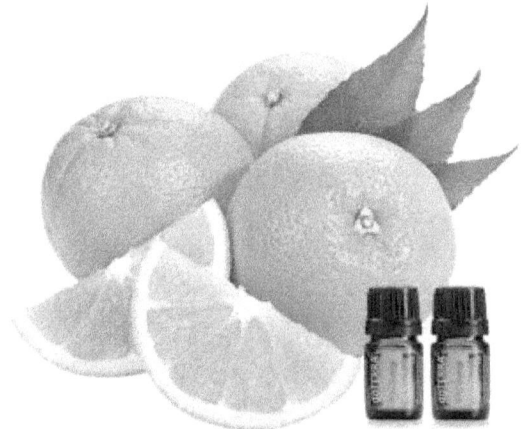

Recipe 04: Immune Booster Blend

Ingredients:

- Melaleuca Essential Oil: 3 Drops
- Oregano Essential Oil: 2 Drops
- Protective Blend: 3 Drops
- Frankincense Essential Oil: 1 Drop
- Carrier Oil: Almond, Jojoba, Etc

Directions:

Before your healthy kids are about to go to bed, a gentle swipe of the blend on the bottom of your child's feet should do the needful. Make sure it's applied regularly before bed for having its effect as an immune booster.

Recipe 05: The Focus Blend For Kids: Great For School-Going Children

Ingredients:

- Peppermint: 3 Drops
- Wild Orange: 3 Drops
- Carrier Oil: Almond, Jojoba, Etc

Directions:

You can apply it on your child's wrist or temples or ask them do it on their own during their school hours. It can be applied on regular intervals throughout the day. It helps staying calm and keep a sharp focus, especially for school-going children.

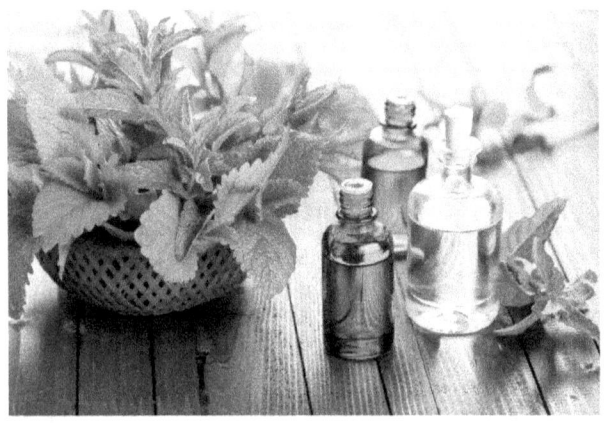

Recipe 06: Roll-On: Anti-Critter

Ingredients:

- Rosemary Essential Oil: 2 Drops
- Melaleuca Essential Oil: 2 Drops
- Eucalyptus Essential Oil: 2 Drops
- Peppermint: 2 Drops
- Carrier Oil: Almond, Jojoba.

Directions:

Roll the mixture on behind the nape of the neck and the ears. It can also be used to roll in your hair and to avoid any bees or wasps from being attracted to the kid's hair. The oil combination has a scent hated by such unwanted guests.

Chapter 2 – DIY Essential Oil Recipes for a Good Night Sleep for All Children

Recipe 07: Good Sleep Boosting Blend:

Ingredients:

- Lemon: 3 Drops
- Oregano: 2 Drops
- Protective Blend: 2 Drops
- Peppermint: 2 Drops
- Clove: 3 Drops
- Melaleuca Essential Oil: 1 Drop
- Carrier Oil: Almond, Jojoba, Etc

Directions:

This powerful essential oil helps your children to get a great sleep at night and wake up as fresh as new the next morning. It would help them get a deep sleep, making them fresh and all set to go the next morning. It can be applied on the child's feet or wrists at night to gain the maximum benefits out of it.

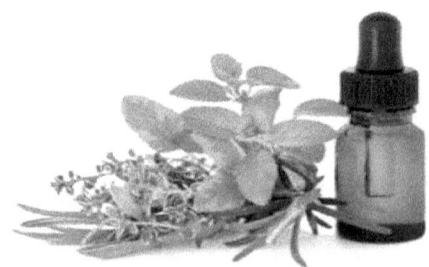

Recipe 8: Super Night Sleep Booster Blend:

Ingredients:

- Melaleuca Essential Oil: 5 Drops
- Oregano: 2 Drops
- Carrier Oil: Almond, Jojoba, Etc
- Protective Blend: 5 Drops
- Frankincense: 2 Drops
- Lemon: 3 Drops

Directions:

This powerful essential oil helps your children to get a great sleep at night and wake up as fresh as new the next morning. It can be applied on the child's feet or wrists at night to gain the maximum benefits out of it. It would help them get a deep sleep, making them fresh and all set to go the next morning.

Recipe 9: Stress Reliever Blend for Kids

Ingredients:

- Peppermint: 8 drops
- Frankincense Essential Oil: 3 drops
- Lavender Essential Oil: 5 drops
- Chamomile Oil: 5 drops
- Carrier Oil: 5 Drops (Almond, Jojoba, Etc)

Directions:

Once the blend is made, it can be applied on the child's nape of neck, forehead and temples. This blend would make sure that your kids get a good deep sleep and wake up relieved with any stress of school or homework.

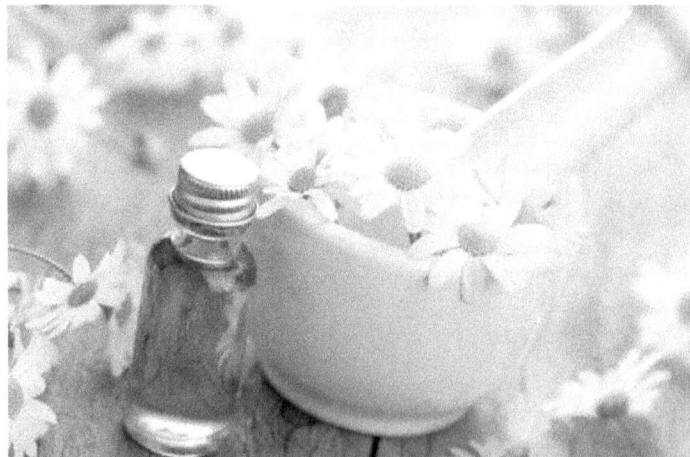

Recipe 10: Sleep Tight – A Good Night Sleep Essential Oil Blend

Ingredients:

- Lavender Essential Oil: 75 Drops
- Sweet Marjoram Essential Oil: 45 Drops
- Roman Chamomile Essential Oil: 30 Drops
- Bergamot Essential Oil: 30 Drops
- Ylang Ylang Essential Oil: 6 Drops
- Valerian Essential Oil: 6 Drops

Directions:

Mix together all the essential oils in a 15 ml bottle and swirl it gently so that all the mixture settles in well with each other. Place a label and keep it in a dark and cool place while not in use with other oils. Your child can use the blend as a smelling salt, aromatherapy inhaler, shower steamers, diffuser in the bedroom or a roll-on. Its proven, your child will have the best sleep ever!

Recipe 11: The Deep Sleep Blend

Ingredients:

- Melaleuca Essential Oil: 1 Drop
- Clove Essential Oil: 3 Drops
- Protective Blend: 2 Drops
- Peppermint Essential Oil: 2 Drops
- Oregano Essential Oil: 2 Drops
- Lemon Essential Oil: 3 Drops
- Carrier Oil: Almond, Jojoba, Etc

Directions:

This blend would make sure that your kids get a good deep sleep and wake up relieved with any stress of school or homework. Mix together all the essential oils in a 15 ml bottle and swirl it gently so that all the mixture settles in well with each other. Once the blend is made, it can be applied on the child's nape of neck, forehead and temples.

Place a label and keep it in a dark and cool place while not in use with other oils. Your child can use the blend as a smelling salt, aromatherapy inhaler, shower steamers, diffuser in the bedroom or a roll-on. It's proven, your child will have the best sleep ever!

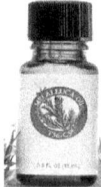

Recipe 12: The Chamomile Sleep Blend:

Ingredients:

- Chamomile Essential Oil: 5 Drops
- Orange Essential Oil: 9 Drops
- Benzoin Essential Oil: 6 Drops
- Moisturizer: 50g

Directions:

Mix these oils well and place them in a bottle. A gentle application on the child's neck and upper chest would help the child sleep deep and is best for kids experiencing nightmares or who frequently get scared.

It's also very effective for kids experiencing insomnia and constipation. It can be used when the kids are bathing and its lovely scent should do the rest while sleeping.

Recipe 13: Cedar wood Calming Recipe

Ingredients:

- Lavender oil – 5 drops
- Cedar wood oil – 5 drops
- Vetiver oil – 5 drops
- Sweet almond oil – 10 drops

Directions:

Get a 5 ml bottle and add the following oils in it such as lavender, cedar wood oil, vetiver oil and sweet almond oil. Blend them together and massage it little on the forehead on your child.

It will keep them calm and they will be able to sleep peacefully with comfort. When they will wake up, they will feel fresh and won't irritate you as much as they used to. Try this and you will be glad that you know this recipe.

Recipe 14: Ylang Ylang Essential Oil Recipe

Ingredients:

- Vetiver – 10 drops
- Lavender – 4 drops
- Ylang Ylang – 4 drops
- Chamomile – 4 drops
- Frankincense oil – 2 drops
- Clary Sage oil – 2 drops
- Marjoram oil – 2 drops
- Coconut oil – 1 tsp.

Directions:

Mix all the ingredients together into a 10 ml bottle. Make sure they all are blend properly and then you can either mix the drop into a diffuser to make it spread all around the house or you can massage your child forehead from it.

This makes an awesome fragrance which you children will surely love so make sure to explain them what it is for and you will see the positive change the next morning.

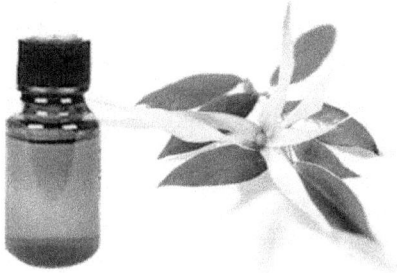

Recipe 15: Mind Calming Blend

Ingredients:

- Frankincense oil – 2 drops
- Pepper mint oil – 3 drops
- Rosemary oil – 4 drops

Directions:

Get a diffuser and add the following ingredients in it such as frankincense oil, pepper mint oil and rosemary oil. Blend it well with the spoon and turn on the diffuser at home.

You will see that you child will be calm and won't be screaming around with disturbing you all the time. it calms their nerves and they are only doing what they want to do without disturbing the mom.

Recipe 16: Lime oil Calming Recipe

Ingredients:

- Peppermint oil – 3 drops
- Lime oil – 4 drops
- Frankincense oil – 4 drops
- Orange essential oil – 6 drops

Directions:

Get a 5 ml bottle and add all the ingredients in it along with water in it. Add peppermint, lime oil, frankincense oil and orange oil together in it. Shake it well and then add the drops into a diffuser. Mix it well.

It will help the child sleep properly without waking up at night again and again. You will see that he/she will be calm than usual.

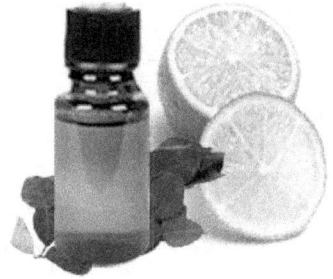

Recipe 17: Grapefruit Calming Recipe

Ingredients:

- Lime oil – 3 drops
- Lemon oil – 5 drops
- Orange oil – 10 drops
- Grapefruit oil – 15 drops
- Lemon grass oil – 10 drops

Directions:

Add all the oils into a 10 ml bottle along with Luke warm bottle. Shake it well and then take the drops in your palm. Blend it in your hand and apply it on your child's forehead. This will help him/her ease up and you will see that their behavior will be changed the next morning when they wake up.

They won't be fussing around much and won't be a pain for you so you can easily use this recipe to keep them calm all day long. Use this regularly and notice the behavior.

Recipe 18: Melissa Oil Recipe

Ingredients:

- Melissa – 10 drops
- Lavender – 10 drops
- Rose – 4 drops

Directions:

Mix all the ingredients in a diffuser and let them spread in the entire house. You do not have to keep your child near it but it will mix into the air which will be inhaled and the child will stay calm. It will keep their head calm and if you wish you can also mix it in a bottle and massage it on their forehead for it to react instantly.

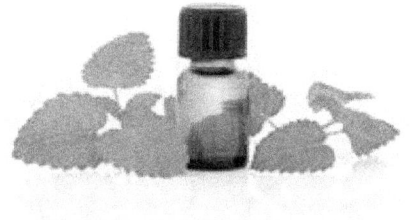

Chapter 4 – Essential Oil Massage Blends for Toddlers

Recipe 19: Sage Oil Massage Recipe for Toddlers

Ingredients:

- Sweet Almond – 10 tbsp.
- Sage – 10 drops
- Marjoram – 5 drops
- Rosemary – 5 drops

Directions:

Get all the ingredients together in the 10 ml bottle and mix them well. After you have mixed them properly then rub it on your hand and massage a little on your toddler body. It will keep the muscles relaxed and they will stay happy most of the times. The essence of essential oils keep their mood light and they do not tend to give you a hard time.

Recipe 20: Bergamot Fun Blend For Massage

Ingredients:

- Lavender oil – 4 drops
- Bergamot oil – 4 drops

Directions:

Mix the ingredients into a 5 ml bottle along with Luke warm water and shake it well. When the mixture is thick and it starts smelling like an essence then lay down your baby and massage the whole body gently.

You will see how happy he/she will get with the massage along with having fun with you.

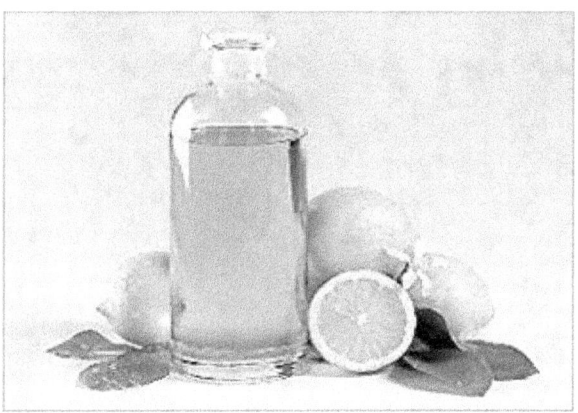

Recipe 21: Juniper Mix Massage Recipe

Ingredients:

- Peppermint – 15 drops
- Black pepper - 15 drops
- Eucalyptus - 15 drops
- Ginger - 15 drops
- Juniper Berry - 15 drops

Directions:

Blend all the ingredients into a bottle and shake it well. Keep it aside for a while and then massage your toddler's forehead with it gently. Make sure that you do it carefully and it does not touch their eyes.

It will have a calming and soothing effect on the baby's body with making them fresh. They won't get lazy and stay active all the time with being engaged with themselves.

Recipe 22: Sweet Almond Mix

Ingredients:

- Sweet Almond
- Rosemary (3 drops)
- Sweet marjoram (4 drops)
- Ginger (1 drop)
- Roman chamomile (6 drops)

Directions:

This is a complete warm body massage for the toddler. Make sure you keep them covered after its application. Mix the ingredients together into a 5 ml bottle along with Luke warm water. Shake it well and then get few drops on your palm.

Massage the whole body of your toddler gently and keep them warm after that for about an hour. It will make them feel easy and relaxed without getting tired and they will not irritate you as well.

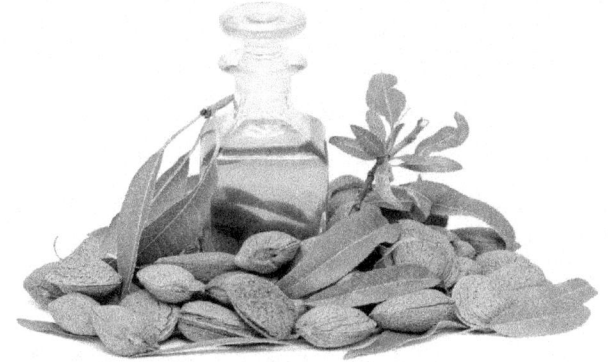

Recipe 23: Coconut oil Massage Therapy

Ingredients:

- Coconut oil (2 tbsp.)
- Sweet marjoram (2 drops)
- Cinnamon (10 drops)
- Peppermint (5 drops)
- Lavender (15 drops)

Directions:

Get a 10 ml bottle and add Luke warm water in it. Mix all the essential oils in it and shake it well. Keep it aside for a while for it settle.

Take some drop and cover your hands with it by applying it on the whole body of your toddler. He/she will feel better and you will see that they won't be crying much as well. They will feel relaxed as long as you are giving them food and staying around them. You can do work in your kitchen and they will be playing on their own without any disturbance.

Recipe 24: Eucalyptus Essential Oil Massage

Ingredients:

- Eucalyptus – 5 drops
- Lavender – 15 drops
- Ginger – 10 drops

Directions:

Get a 5 ml bottle and these essential oils drops in it. Shake it well and then add Luke warm water in it. Keep it aside for about an hour and then massage the forehead of your baby with this. You can massage the feet bottom with it as well to give the relaxing feel to the baby to take away their tiredness. You will see that they will fall asleep within some time because they will feel relaxed and easy on their head.

Sometimes the babies irritate because they want parents to be with them all the time but this massage will help them stay normal even if you are doing your house chores and he/she is playing on his own.

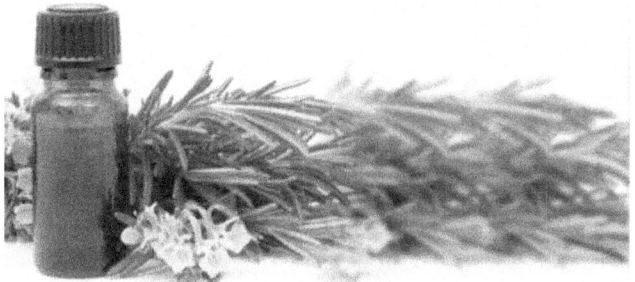

Chapter 5 – Essential Oil Blends to Protect Children from Allergies and Infections

Recipe 25: Clove Recipe Blend for Allergy

Ingredients:

- Clove – 2 drops
- Lavender – 3 drops
- Peppermint – 3 drops
- Birch – 2 drops
- Thyme – 2 drops

Directions:

Mix all the ingredients in a bowl and add them into a diffuser. Turn on the diffuser at night time or when you wake up in the morning which will be inhaled by the children. It will help them decrease the allergies and they won't be having any headaches or pains.

Recipe 26: Ginger Magic Blend

Ingredients:

- Marjoram – 15 drops
- Lavender – 15 drops
- Ginger – 10 drops
- Rosemary – 15 drops

Directions:

Add all the ingredients in a 5 ml bottle and shake it well. Keep it aside to settle and then add it into a diffuser for the essence to spread all around the house. This will help your child stay away from the bacteria and infections which they can catch.

The essence is inhaled and causes the body to heal and remove any bacteria from the body by flushing it out and giving a rest to the brain as well.

Recipe 27: Yarrow Oil Blend

Ingredients:

- Yarrow – 3 drops
- Clove oil – 10 drops
- Peppermint – 10 drops

Directions:

The yarrow oil helps to relieve allergies quickly so add it with clove oil and peppermint oil in a 5 ml bottle and shake it well. Turn on the diffuser and add the drops into it to have the essence spread in the house.

When the essence is inhaled, it helps to keep the children calm from fussing if they are not feeling well and also heals then inside with the treatment of natural ingredients.

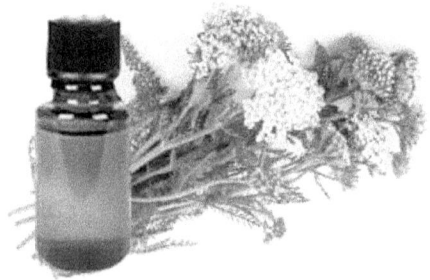

Recipe 28: Black Pepper Blend

Ingredients:

- Ginger – 20 drops
- Cinnamon – 12 drops
- Black pepper – 12 drops

Directions:

Black pepper is the best for the allergies to calm so add them with ginger and cinnamon in a 10 ml bottle by shaking it well. You can use it both ways by massing it over the forehead of your child gently or by adding the drops into the diffuser.

Recipe 29: Cypress Remedy Blend

Ingredients:

- Sweet Almond – 14 tbsp.
- Sweet marjoram – 20 drops
- Cypress – 12 drops
- Ginger – 4 drops

Directions:

Add all the ingredients in a 10 ml bottle with Luke warm water in it. Mix them well by shaking the bottle thoroughly. When done, add the drops into the diffuser to help you child get some relieve from the allergies.

The healing power of the essential oils helps the nerves to calm down and fixes any infection which is minor without any further step.

Recipe 30: Sweet Marjoram Recipe

Ingredients:

- Roman chamomile – 10 drops
- Sweet marjoram – 5 drops
- Lavender oil – 3 drops

Directions:

Mix all the ingredients in a bottle and shake them well. Make sure that you keep it aside for a while for the oils to blend in each other. It works as the best treatment for the child who is sneezing all day long. Gives a warm feel when inhaled through the diffuser.

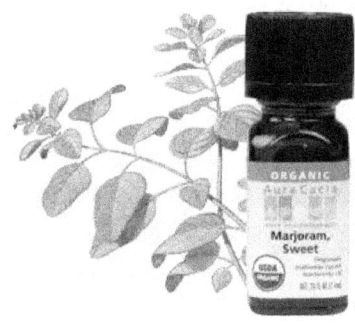

Conclusion

If you are someone who is new to the world of essential oils, then it is better to start with the lighter ones. The fragrance may seem too strong in the beginning if you jump to the clove scent because it is strong and may be a reason for your headache at one point. A list of all the possible blends is available for you in the eBook which is easy to make. You simply need to have the water and add the oils in it. There is no proper direction for each but the similar procedure for you to follow.

The essential oils fragrance works like magic for those who stay stress from their busy lives and makes your pains go away. Life becomes tough, and we tend to forget how actually to manage it so then comes the main role of the essential oils which soothes your brain and gives you some peace to your kids. You can relax and massage on your child's body easily at any time with the essential oils blends.

It depends on the size of the jar in which you are making the blends but mostly people try the small ones, and the instructions are based on that also. You can try any of these recipes at your home, and you will see how peaceful it will be. They work wonders and keeps your child calm in your daily life routine without any disturbance. Once you start liking the essence of it, you will be glad that you have this eBook to try other new blends. This eBook is full of awesome recipes to try on your kids which are safe and will always have a positive effect on your kids.